7 Day Ultimate Detox Cleanse: Lose Weight and Revitalize Your Life

In 7 Days or Less Experience the Complete Detox Cleanse

By: Marlo Walken

PUBLISHERS NOTES

This publication is intended to provide helpful and informative material. It is not intended to diagnose, treat, cure, or prevent any health problem or condition, nor is intended to replace the advice of a physician. No action should be taken solely on the contents of this book. Always consult your physician or qualified health-care professional on any matters regarding your health and before adopting any suggestions in this book or drawing inferences from it.

The author and publisher specifically disclaim all responsibility for any liability, loss or risk, personal or otherwise, which is incurred as a consequence, directly or indirectly, from the use or application of any contents of this book.

Any and all product names referenced within this book are the trademark of their respective owners. None of these owners have sponsored, authorized, endorsed, or approved this book.

Always read all information provided by the manufacturers' product labels before using their products. The author and publisher are not responsible for claims made by manufacturers.

Trade Paperback Edition

Manufactured in the United States of America

What You Will Learn In This Book

How This Book Will Help You and Why

The idea behind a detoxification diet is to improve circulation in the blood, eliminate toxins stored in blood, improve digestion, reduce stress on the body, and promote overall mind and body wellness.

There are several factors that cause the body to operate inefficiently, and detoxification attempts to eliminate these factors and repair internal systems through good foods.

This book will walk you through the process of doing a complete detox not just the ordinary everyday detox.

ABOUT THE AUTHOR

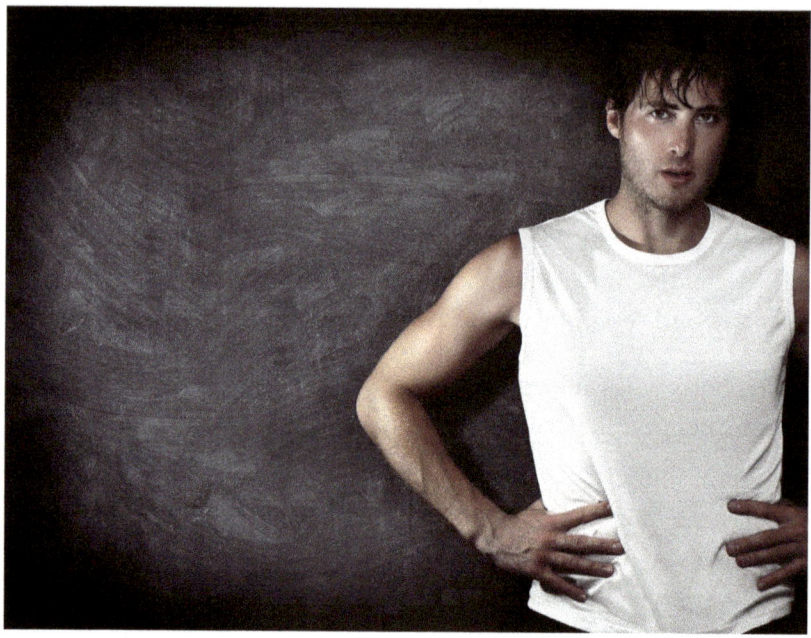

Marlo Walken literally got a new lease on life when he had his first detox and he has not looked back since then. He was overweight, sickly and unhappy. He modified his diet and started to exercise but still found that he still lacked something.

He tried the 7 day detail cleanse and has not had a bad day since then. His body got the reboot that it needed and he was able to complete his weight loss journey and maintain his new healthier weight.

In his book he outlines what the detox cleanse is and who it is best suited for. He also cites a lot of his personal experiences in the book. He highlights throughout that it is a jumpstart to a healthier lifestyle and that other changes have to be made to make it all worthwhile. The book is both informative and educational.

TABLE OF CONTENTS

Publishers Notes	2
What You Will Learn In This Book	3
About The Author	4
Table of Contents	6
What Celebrities Have To Say	7
What Is The Detox Diet	8
Let's Get Started With Master Cleanse	11
Try The Liver Detox	15
THE FOOT DETOX HOW DOES IT WORK	19
COLON CLEANSE & DETOX	22
HEAVY METAL DETOX	26
SUGAR DETOX – THE BEST STEP	29
PARASITE CLEANSE AND DETOX	32
DETOX RECIPES	36
WATER DETOX MADE EASY	51

WHAT CELEBRITIES HAVE TO SAY

"A systemic cleansing and detox is definitely the way to go after each holiday. It is the key to fighting high blood pressure, heart disease, cancer, and other health-related illnesses."

- Lee Haney

WHAT IS THE DETOX DIET

A detoxification diet generally is a short term healing diet lasting 7-21 days which restricts processed foods, dairy, and fried foods. It increases fruits and vegetables, and cleanses the body of harmful toxins that may have built up in the body from chemicals, processed foods and other agents.

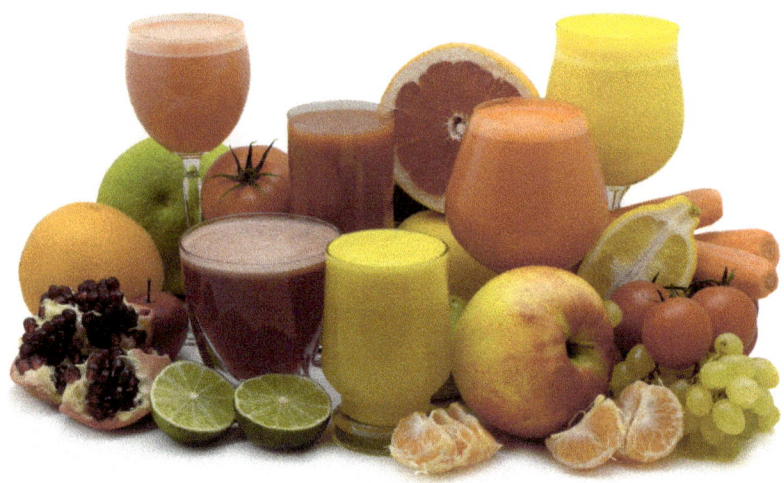

It creates healthy functioning of internal organs, reduces inflammation, and brings the body back into PH balance, promoting more effective weight loss.

Not only does such a diet prepare the body for weight loss, but the primary function of a detoxification diet is to improve bodily functions and remove agents causing organs and internal systems to improperly function. This is thought to improve overall good health. It also removes potential barriers to good health and weight control.

The idea behind a detoxification diet is to improve circulation in the blood, eliminate toxins stored in blood, improve digestion, reduce stress on the body, and promote overall mind and body wellness.

There are several factors that cause the body to operate inefficiently, and detoxification attempts to eliminate these factors and repair internal systems through good foods.

Problems in blood circulation can lead to many problems, including disease. Improper diets can affect the blood, as can lack of exercise. By eliminating processed foods, and introducing foods good for the cardiovascular system, such as green leafy vegetables this promotes healing. Detoxification, coupled with an exercise program, can stimulate healing.

Another detoxification issue is the toxins that are stored in the cells. These cells enter the blood and cause many health problems. By eliminating the toxins through increased water intake, lemons and other foods toxins are naturally removed through the waste process.

This allows for the body to return to proper functioning, and prevents future health problems associated with free radicals and lack of antioxidants in the body.

Proper digestion is a concern in all weight loss programs, and detoxification seeks to repair digestion issues. This is done by introducing good bacteria into the intestines through foods such as yogurt, and nutrient rich foods.

Eating foods that eliminate bad bacteria such as garlic, turmeric, and green leafy vegetables help to promote good health. Lack of good bacteria in the intestines not only causes digestion problems, but injures the cell membranes of the body, leading to future health problems.

The introduction of nutrient rich foods during detoxification promotes the growth of good bacteria. As this occurs digestion and liver functions improves. Wheat gluten is eliminated during detoxification, and increased liver functions occur due to increased amounts of proteins, nutrients, vitamins, and foods containing high levels of antioxidants.

Another issue related to improper body functions and detoxification is stress placed on the body with diets high in processed foods and fatty carbohydrates. High sugar, high carbohydrate, high fat diets lead to a myriad of health problems.

By eliminating these agents from diets digestive and immune system functions improve. As the body's functions improve stress on the body and its organs is removed and an overall feeling of body, mind and spirit wellness occurs.

Detoxification foods include green vegetables, especially leafy greens and spinach. Other foods good for detoxification are lemons, limes, broccoli, green tea, nuts, omega oils, cauliflower and cabbage.

These foods, and others, help bring the body back into proper balance, increase health and reduce harmful toxins from the body. As nutrients and anti-oxidants in the body increase, and sugars, and processed foods decrease overall health improves.

In addition to healing detoxification foods drink plenty of water and introduce healing green tea into diets, which is full of antioxidants, regulates blood sugar, and may prevent cancer and other diseases.

LET'S GET STARTED WITH MASTER CLEANSE

DAY 1 – START THE MASTER CLEANSE

Magazines, T.V. shows, and major celebrities have all spilled their secret weapon for health and fast weight loss: The Master Cleanse.

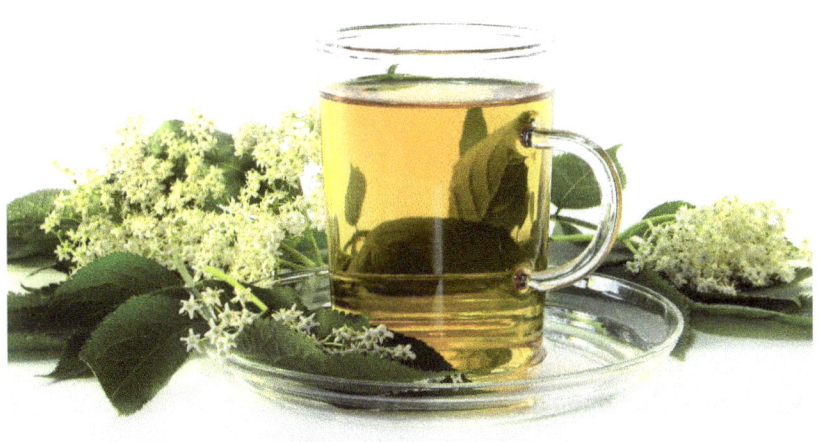

The Master Cleanse is a structured fasting plan that originated in 1940. Since then, millions have reported huge weight loss, higher energy, mental clarity, and have sworn that ailments they were experiencing have healed.

The theory behind the Master Cleanse is that by allowing your body to rest and not have to digest and process food- particularly processed foods, you allow your body time to heal itself from other occurring ailments. During the process you will also purge all toxins and chemicals out of your body. Most references indicate that the

Master Cleanse should be used for a minimum of 10 days with a proper 'ease-in' and 'ease-out' stage. Some say the diet should be used for a maximum of 40 consecutive days, but that you may repeat the Master Cleanse several times throughout the year.

How do you use it?

The Master Cleanse has a series of 3 steps: The ease-in, the lemonade diet, and the ease out phase. The Ease-in phase allows your body 3 days to get used to not having foods and allows you to emotionally prepare for the difficulty of fasting over several days (or for some, several weeks). The Lemonade Diet phase is where most of the weight loss and detoxing effects will occur.

For at least 10 days you will only drink a lemonade mixture of fresh lemon juice, cayenne pepper, purified water and maple syrup, allowing your body enough daily nutrients, but shedding the unwanted toxins and fat from your body. The Ease out phase entails reintroducing solids to your body so that you may continue to make healthy life choices after your cleanse.

Another key component to making sure that all toxins are released and that your body is properly maintained, is the colon cleansing addition. Clearing your bowels can be achieved with either a saltwater mix drink, or with the help of a laxative tea.

Below are the details:

Phase 1: <u>The Ease-In</u>

You should consider the kind of diet you would like to maintain once you are finished with the Master Cleanse. The Master Cleanse is but a vehicle for you to start new. Day 1 of easing in should be focused on whole food choices and all meat, dairy, and processed foods must be eliminated.

Eat a balance between fruits and vegetables. Day 2 should focus on water-based foods like soup, broths, and juices. This phase will get your body used to a liquid diet. Day 3 you only drink orange juice. The carbohydrates of orange juice will keep you energetic while your body adjusts to the changes.

Phase 1.5: Decide which method of bowel cleansing is right for you. You can either

A. take an herbal laxative at night and in the morning or B. Take an herbal laxative at night and do a saltwater rinse in the morning or C. Do the saltwater rinse at night and the laxative in the morning. Finding the right amount of laxatives for your body is a process. If there is no bowel movement, you can scale up the amount taken. If your bowl movement is immediate and does not ensure a night's sleep, scale down a bit.

Phase 2: <u>The Lemonade Diet</u>

Each day you should drink 6-12 glasses of lemonade. Each glass should contain the following:

2 tablespoons **<u>Lemon Juice</u>**

2 tablespoons of **<u>Maple Syrup</u>**

Pinch of **<u>Cayenne Pepper</u>**

8 oz. of **<u>Purified Water</u>**.

Phase 2.5: Each night take a laxative or do the Saltwater Rinse. The Saltwater Rinse consists of a quart of purified water and 2 teaspoons of Sea Salt. You must 'chug' the mixture, preferably in one sitting. You must do this on an empty stomach and when you are free to eliminate within the next half an hour. Make sure you set aside time to be able to make a bowel movement after drinking this, as it will occur.

Phase 3: Ease-Out phase

The ease out phase is to help your body readjust to a solid diet. Simply follow the ease-in phase instructions from end to beginning.

Good luck cleansing and making the transition to a healthy lifestyle.

TRY THE LIVER DETOX

DAY 2 – GRADUALLY EASE INTO THE LIVER DETOX

Liver detox dieting has become a pressing health topic in cyberspace. Society has learned the dangers of liver intoxication. Today, physicians and their patients have teamed together to find natural solutions. The main concern is to limit the risk factors.

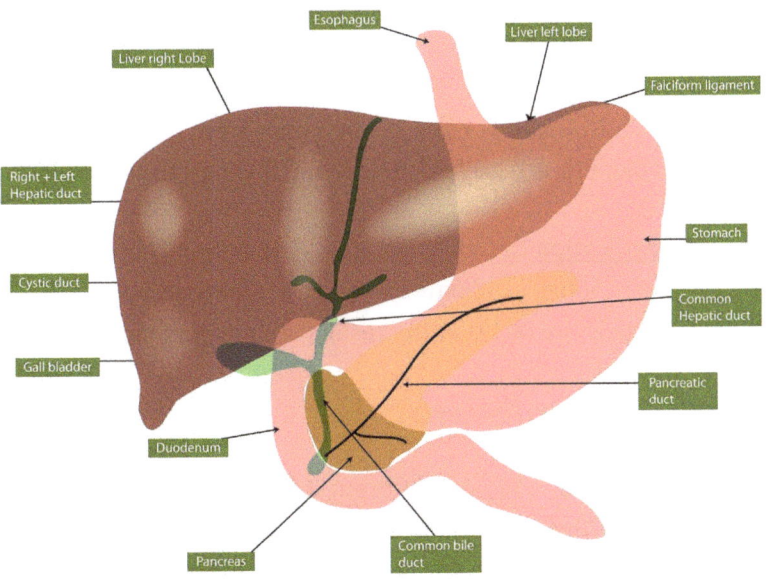

Liver Detoxification Explained

Liver cleansing is the process of removing harmful toxins in the organ and body. There's an ample selection of methods that offer appreciable results. Natural diets that focus on liver detoxification give permanent relief. Medical programs also extend solutions that work.

How do Liver Detox Solutions Work

The liver itself carries out a series of detoxification tasks in the body. It is an elemental activity to protect the core processes. If the liver is not functioning at an optimal level, it exposes the body to health risks. Efficient liver cleansing solutions remedy underlying problems that slow down productivity in the body.

The first stage of the liver detox process involves fasting/purging the organ. With the inclusion of a disciplined diet that includes nourishing foods and nutrients, it is possible to restore balance.

Two days is enough time to rid the body of toxic waste through fasting. Salads, water, Epsom salts and fresh juices, including lemon, apple, etc. are exceptional for the fasting/purging regime.

<u>**Liver detoxification**</u> has many variants. The option chosen depends on the host. Some candidates opt for a synthetic approach. The disadvantage is the fact that the results are not permanent.

Benefits of detoxing the liver

Toxins enter the body in different forms. Caffeine, pesticides, smog, air pollution, medications, impure water, alcohol, sugar and a variety of other foods are conduits that export toxins into the body. Liver detoxification has numerous health benefits.

A diet focused on liver detox can help to revitalize the body. In addition, it is an efficacious method of improving the skin appearance, digestion and concentration. There have been studies that report weight loss achievement and increased energy as well.

The best way to aid the liver to improve the biological detoxification process is to consume nutrient-rich foods to support the organs. The liver has two core processing segments. The first phase converts the toxins into free radicals, which is a less harmful property.

Unfortunately, this molecule of articles need sufficient amounts of antioxidants. This is to slow down their activity and prevent cell damage. The second stage involves a process where the body gets rid of metabolic waste, including free radicals. The kidney and colon are the key waste-processing organs.

List of top 5 liver detox foods

Garlic

Grapefruit

Carrots/Beets

Green Tea

Leafy Green Vegetables

EFFICIENT LIVER DETOX RECIPE: BEET JUICE

Beet juice is an essential, liver boosting supplement. With the right ingredients, toxic liver victims will experience the energy-boosting effects.

Ingredients

1 beet

1 carrot

1 lemon, peeled

1 handful of parsley

Directions

Put all the ingredients in a blender or juicer.

Puree the mixture at a moderate speed.

Remove it from the container once the process has been completed.

Store the mixed beverage in the refrigerator and drink as needed.

Cleansing the liver of impurities has advantages and disadvantages. A rule to liver detox is to detect the body's natural signs and symptoms to know when it warrants cleansing.

Some common examples of lifestyle habits that result in liver intoxication, includes restlessness, low energy, poor supply of nutrients, over exercising and heavy alcohol consumption.

Toxins overtax the liver when the body has excessive amounts. This spreads to other organs and causes permanent/temporary damages.

The liver is an organ that is usually ignored until emergency health problems arise. Physicians are putting emphasis on patient education to reduce the risk of liver damages and other organ diseases.

The liver undertakes essential functions to keep the body active, sustainable and healthy. It needs the right nutrients to keep performance at optimal levels.

THE FOOT DETOX HOW DOES IT WORK

DAY 3 – BEGIN THE PROCESS OF THE FOOT DETOX

Over time the body builds up toxins from pollution, poor diet, chemicals, and normal bodily functions – *But can the feet work?*

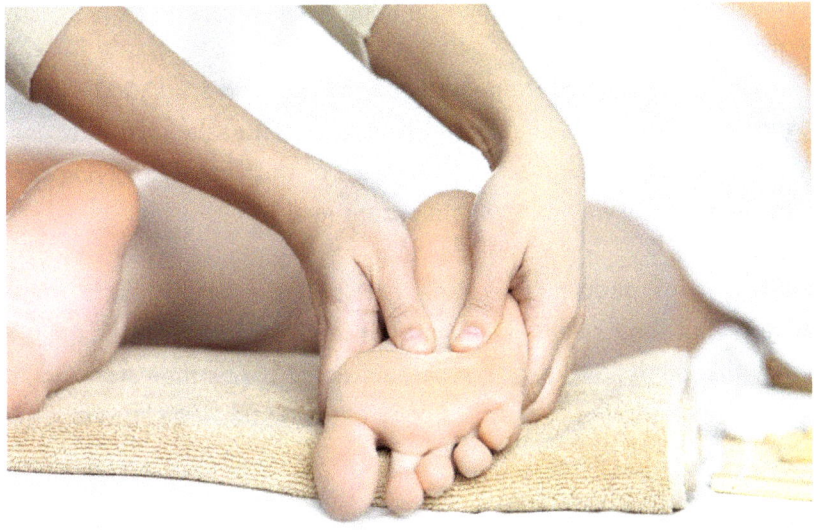

In order to maintain optimum health, cleansing the body through diet and detoxification is important. There are many ways to detoxify the body from colon cleansing and detox diets to total dietary changes and fasting.

Because the body is a storehouse of what people put in it, and much of what we put in it can prove toxic to the body or is waste it is important to cleanse and purge the body frequently.

Many people understand some of the basics of detoxifying certain parts of the body, but the whole body has areas where it takes in toxins including the skin which is the body's largest organ.

One of the areas of the body that is inclined to build up toxins is the foot. Since much of the body has glands such as the underarm and groin area, it should be of no surprise to learn that the feet have many glands that can house toxins as well.

In fact, **the feet contain between 250,000 and 300,000 sweat glands**. That means that each gland area can easily take in toxins especially as a person sweats. Because of this foot detoxifying can be an essential way to maintain proper health.

While many people know their feet sweat, many others do not know that their sweat glands in their feet can actually also clog up and this can lead to health problems as the toxins then store up in the body. The partial purpose of sweating is to purge the body of toxins.

That in part is why many natural health doctors recommend saunas and sweat baths as a way to cleanse the body. This natural sweating gets rid of toxins in the feet as well.

Through the help and assistance of detoxification cleansers the foot glands of a person can help people to find a better way to purge the body of the build-up of toxins.

There are several ways to detox the sweat glands of the body through the feet. There are detoxifying foot baths, detoxifying foot pads and detoxifying foot washes.

No matter what type of detoxifying process is chosen the most important thing to consider is the ingredients used. Most often if the ingredients are all natural they will be helpful, but this is not always the case.

Some of the best all natural ingredients that people are familiar with for foot detoxification are Oatmeal, Baking Soda and Epsom salts.

But there are other ingredients that can readily be found in the home as well, two of these are teas. Both Peppermint Tea and Chamomile Tea are great for a foot soak detoxifying. Another foot soak is honey and lemon.

Lemon is a natural astringent and Honey is a natural antibiotic. As with any natural use of honey, local honey is best because the properties of the honey are not processed and over refined into a less potent form.

There are foot detoxifying machines that are also quite helpful and can be used with many of these home remedies to thoroughly purge the body of the built up toxins in the foot glands.

For people who have been using cleaning products, or who have had recent X-rays, have been ill or have had exposure to chemicals, using a foot detoxifying bath is a good way of purging some of those toxins out of the body.

The process need not be a lengthy one. A simple 15 minute soak, bath or wash can prove to be quite helpful in detoxifying the body.

COLON CLEANSE & DETOX

DAY 4 – START WITH COLON CLEANSING

Ancient Egyptians held the belief that putrefied feces line the walls of the large intestine and when these accumulate it causes parasites (pathogenic flora) to grow resulting in general ill health. Whereas, this theory was eventually discredited in the early 20th century, some people, today, still practice modern colon cleansing.

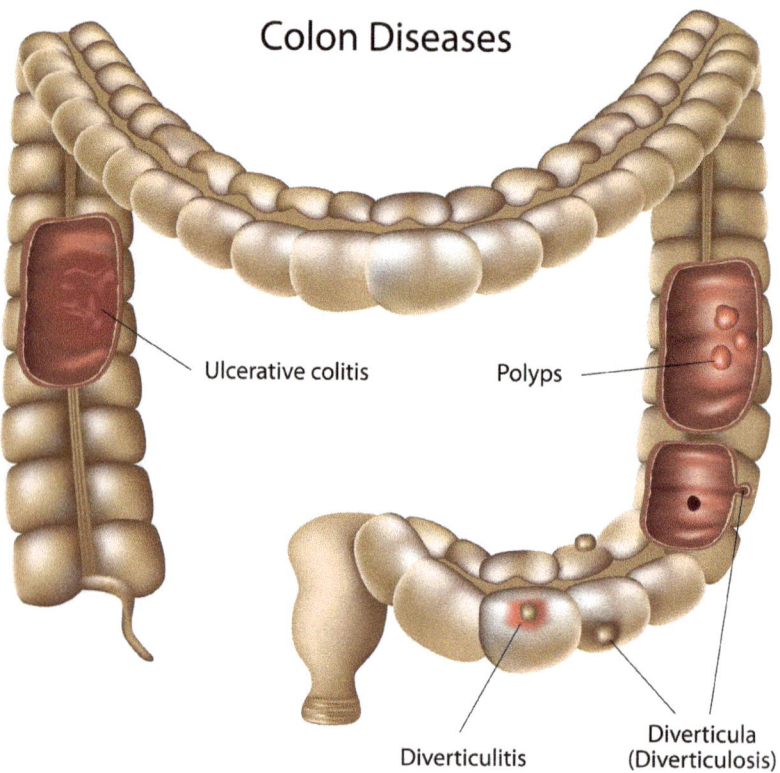

The "auto-intoxication" belief, so dearly, held up by the ancient civilizations, claimed that headaches, loss of appetite, irritability and fatigue were results of it. As modern science was born, it dispelled with these ideas stating that according to medical fact these symptoms were being caused by mechanical distention within the bowels.

Additionally, the therapies associated with these were based on rather vaguely promoted concepts by certain manufacturers in order to sell cleansing products. At one time it was considered big business.

There are several names that are synonymous with colon cleansing, such as hydrotherapy or colonic irrigation. Although there is no scientific evidence to support the fact that colon cleansing works or does what it is targeted to do, there are quite a few products available to do it.

It was in the early part of this century that infomercials and internet marketing increased promotions of oral supplements that would be beneficial to colon detox.

Among the many ways that colon cleansing is achieved, two methods are increasingly popular, hydrotherapy and oral regimens. The hydrotherapy method uses tubular equipment to inject water mixed with supplements or herbs via the rectum. The oral method promotes diets based on dietary fiber, herbs, supplements and laxatives.

Doctors all over the world are now actively countering this by explaining that nature already does great job of waste disposal. They go on to say that procedures based on these hydro-therapies may cause damage to the rectum.

Additionally, there is increasing evidences that some enema preparations risk electrolyte imbalance and carries the risk of heart attacks. They go on to point out that poorly maintained equipment can cause infection and improperly used equipment may damage the bowels,

Hydro-therapies have increasingly become questionable because scientists point out that hydrotherapy causes to disrupt the natural flora of the human intestinal tract resulting in electrolyte depletion or even dehydration.

Medical records have even been recorded for far more adverse events such as rectal perforation and amoebic infections. Some even say that these colon cleansing procedures impede in the colon's natural ability to shed dead cells.

Hydrotherapy is a process described as the injection of water, through the rectum, into the colon. This is then held for 15 minutes. The solution may be just water or a mixture of water with herbs. This process is repeated till the colon is considered washed out.

Colon detox is best described as an oral method where one a single scoop of colon detoxify powder is mixed with 8 ounces of diluted juice and consumed in a day. This process typically lasts 30 days. Along with this you must also take a colon corrective formula to avoid constipation.

There have been reported cases of severe constipation even while ingesting a colon corrective formula. Other supplements used in oral detoxification are laxatives, magnesium, herbal teas and enzymes. Various manufacturers promote their products by stating the effectiveness of one type over another.

It is a well-known fact that doctors prescribe colon cleansing as a prelude to a medical procedure known as a colonoscopy, but do not recommend the cleansing for the purposes of detoxification.

Proponents of colon detoxification claim that various health issues such as arthritis, certain allergies and even asthma, can be resolved through this process. They additionally claim that this boosts your immune system and increases energy.

HEAVY METAL DETOX

DAY 5 – DROP IN THE HEAVY METAL DETOX

Mercury, lead, and aluminium are all heavy metals that collect in the body over time. These heavy metals are thought to cause heart disease, thyroid problems, dementia, birth defects, infertility, autism, and neurological conditions. But, there is a way to remove these from your body using heavy metal detoxification.

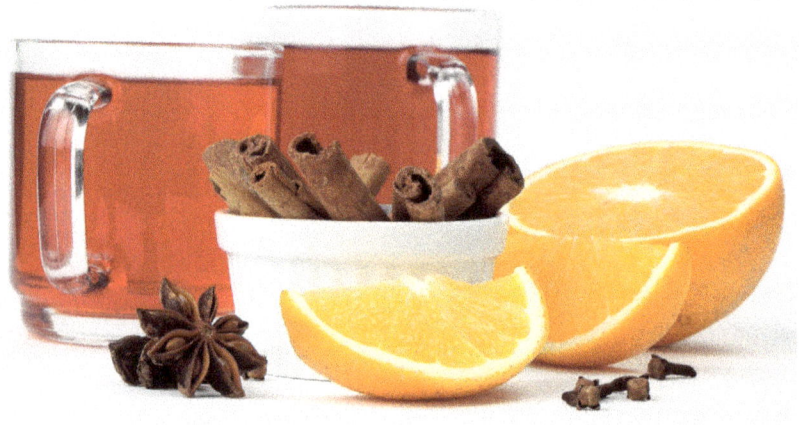

Heavy metal detoxification is a process where metals are put in the body from thing like drugs, and is treated by detoxing the body through heavy metal detoxification. During heavy metal detoxification people change their diet, and daily routine slightly to help rid their bodies of the harmful metals that are currently in their bodies.

In Heavy Metal detoxification people limit the amount of mercury that they intake. This detoxification recommends eating fish eating significantly less mercury. Mercury amalgam tooth filling can contribute to the amount of mercury in the body as well.

Some people get these fillings replaced to eliminate that problem. When getting vaccinated it is recommended to ask for mercury free vaccines. Some vaccines still contain mercury based preservative thimersal.

Clean the water! Water contains pollution just as much as air does. Pollution contains a lot of harmful heavy metals. So it is suggested to drink filtered water. Paint before the 1970's contained a lot of lead. If you work or live in an older building chances are there is lead based paint.

Cilantro is yummy! Cilantro is a natural chelating agent. There are many ways to eat it to. You can put it in pesto, pasta, toast, and spaghetti. Other leafy greens and vegetables are fantastic to eat as well. Along with plenty of fruits!

Detox diets are there to rid your body of heavy metals and toxins. When done correctly will ensure long lasting benefits, and the natural cleansing of your body.

Bad eating habits can result in arthritis. Doctors recommend consuming less caffeine, and nonorganic produce. Cleansing your body is a great way to detox heavy metals. The heavy metal detox does this in a natural way.

Drinking a lot of water helps with this as water is a natural cleanser in itself. Start eating raw fruits and vegetables! This is very nutritious, and great for getting essential nutrients for your body. Try and cut out dairy, grains consisting gluten, meat, and shellfish. Also, processed foods, artificial sweeteners, and sugars are great to avoid as well.

Heavy metal detox eliminates heavy metals, and is also great for getting essential vitamins and minerals for the body. Carrots, broccoli, citrus, avocado, oranges, bananas, and leafy greens are fantastic sources of vitamins and minerals essential to the body. Herbs and spices are also good ways to remove toxins from the body.

Herbs and spices also help with the body's digestion. Some herbs and spices are found to have amazing antioxidant and anti-inflammatory properties. These are great for the body's immune system when sick, or just to boost your immune system. Herbs and spices are excellent for detoxing the body as well as boosting the body's immune system.

Try and keep the detox diet.

A natural (nothing extreme) detox diet will help your body naturally detox itself continuously. Which will result in better health for your body. Your body will thank your someday for doing the heavy metal detox. If you stay with the heavy metal detox diet then your body will continuously detox itself. Just make sure that it is nothing extreme.

The detox diet uses natural detoxes such as water, and detoxing foods to naturally detox the body of all the harmful toxins and heavy metals in the body. This will result boosting your bodies' health.

Sugar Detox – The best Step

DAY 6 – CUT OUR SUGAR FOR THE NEXT 21 DAYS

Sugar is one of the leading factors for obesity, diabetes and other health problems in America, aside from fast food. The country centers all their food around one ingredient and that is sugar.

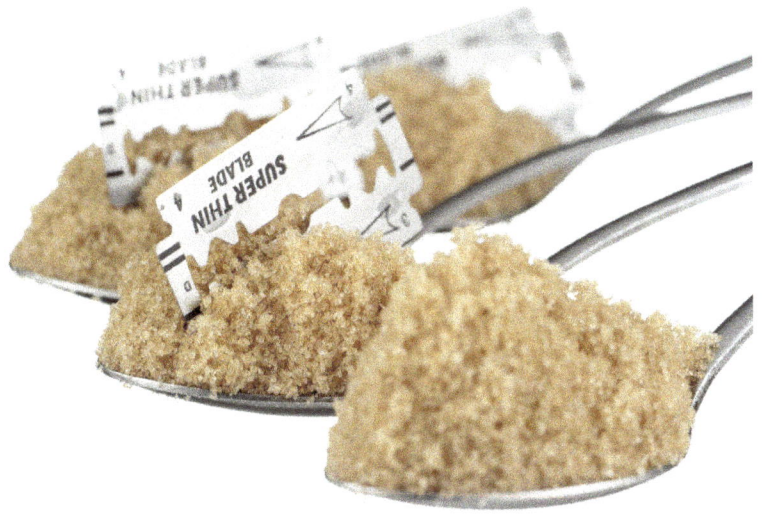

This country has more obese people than any other country in the world. It is said by many professionals that a person will consume about 70 lbs of sugar each year. A diet this high in sugar leads to health problems such heart disease and type II diabetes. The solution is to control sugar intake or eliminate it completely from one's diet.

To begin eliminating or reducing the amount of sugar in one's diet, it would be important to start with a sugar detox.

Now you are probably wondering what a sugar detox is. A sugar detox just like any other detox is going through a time period approximately 21 days where you eliminate sugar from your diet cold turkey and begin a new way of eating, this will expel the toxin build-up from your body.

The detox period is the time frame where your body will adjust to not having any type of sugar entering your body; so that you may naturally cleanse your body of all the sugar it has consumed. You should think of this as an addiction as you would with drugs or alcohol; when you detox you are getting the substance out of your body. This is where you are trying to begin a new eating lifestyle without the need or cravings of sugars.

The way it works is that each day you will create a menu for all your meals and snacks. You will begin loading yourself up with protein and fiber and eliminating starchy foods and sugars. Think of it as spring cleaning of the body; when you spring clean your house you get rid of "wastes", this is the same thing you will do when you do the detox.

You will substitute different foods and snacks in place of what you would normally eat. For example, instead of going for a candy bar in the afternoon; you can have some nuts, celery or a hard-boiled egg. You are training your body to reach for protein and fiber, not sugar.

After the initial 21 days, it will be second nature to change the way you eat. You can have a bowl of unsweetened oatmeal with fruit to give it flavor or an apple with peanut butter.

These are healthier alternatives to those sugary products that your body was used to. Removing the sugar from your diet will allow you to eat what your body needs and get a sense of being satisfied instead of overeating and allowing the sugar to convert to fat.

Once you are out of your detox period then you will slowly introduce natural sugars back into your diet. The detox allows you to get rid of the toxins that were clogging up your body and you can start all over. Just remember that you will have to be sure not to exceed the recommended dosage of sugar per day, so it would be best to start with small amounts.

By eliminating the sugars from your diet, you are rejuvenating your body; this means you will no longer feel tired and sluggish and your skin and body will begin to reap the benefits of being healthy.

The detoxing removes toxins and wastes from your body and replaces it with vital nutrients that your body needs. It is important to do the detox in order to start fresh with your body. The first few days are the hardest but after that, it should just come naturally.

PARASITE CLEANSE AND DETOX

DAY 7 – BEGIN THE PROCESS OF THE PARASITE CLEANSE

Our bodies are susceptible to parasites even when we do not know it. There are many ways in which parasites get into our bodies. Dirty water contains a lot of contaminants as well as parasites. Food that is not properly cooked also hides a lot of parasites.

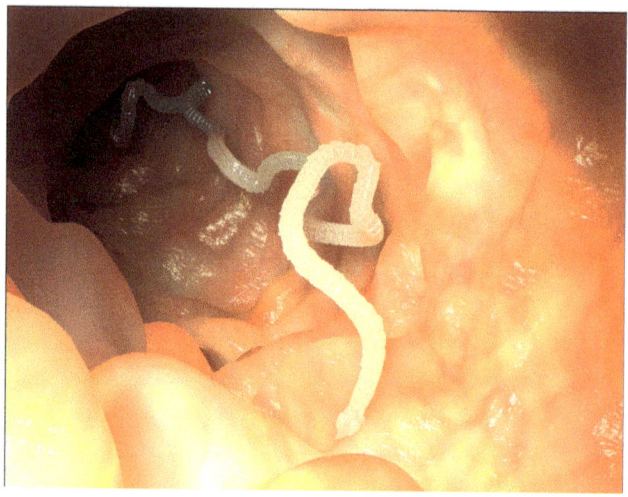

You may be exposed to parasites through poor hygiene. When parasites inhabit, they will feed off of nutrients meant for the body.

They will also reproduce and excrete toxins that eventually cause illness. Common symptoms caused by parasites include: gas, bloating, diarrhea, headaches, irritable bowel syndrome, skin rashes, cravings and even acne. Parasites will also cause fatigue in some cases. So what is parasite cleansing and detox?

Parasite cleansing and detox encompasses all activities that help get rid of parasites from your body as well as cleanse your digestive system. After this process is done, you will feel a lot better both inside and out. Here is what you want to do in order to clean your system.

The first step in parasite cleansing and detox is to practice good personal hygiene. Our hands are exposed to a lot of germs even from surfaces and places that we might not think of. This is why it is very important to make sure you are constantly washing your hands.

Cleansing can either be carried out naturally or in extreme cases through medication. However, it does not have to get to that point. Cleansing and detoxification should be done regularly to get rid of parasites and to also remain healthy.

Start by going on a diet that weakens parasites in your body. Garlic is highly recommended for this. You can take raw garlic with your meals every day for about a week. Foods that help in cleansing the body include fruits, leafy green vegetables, whole grains, and nuts.

Foods with a lot of fiber will help you have regular bowel movements therefore helping to remove toxins from your body. Eat nuts raw without frying them and without salts.

With fruits you have to be extra careful, since you do not want to eat too much sugar, or worsen the situation by eating unwashed fruit. The best approach is to choose one fruit and eat it regularly for a week or so.

Apples are a good choice. You may also use few drops of lemon juice or oregano oil in drinking water. These have very powerful anti-parasitic properties.

Herbs are also effective in parasite cleansing and detox. Cloves, wormwood and black walnut powder are some of the most effective parasite killers. Other effective remedies include pumpkin seeds, extra virgin coconut oil, Neem and turmeric.

As you cleanse, it is important to maintain a high fiber diet and drink plenty of water. There are also pills and herbal extracts sold by chemists that can also help you cleanse. Regular de-worming pills are crucial in keeping off parasites from your system. Medication may be necessary at some point to counteract toxins released when parasites die.

It is also important to avoid junk food and eat fresh natural food as much as possible. Cleansing will keep you healthy by ensuring regular bowel movements hence keeping your digestive system healthy and reducing any risks of colon cancer. Cleansing is also known to cause an increase in energy.

When you feel energized it is a lot easier to do regular exercise which also helps you do cleanse and detox. You want to sweat as much as possible to release even more toxins that are built up inside your body.

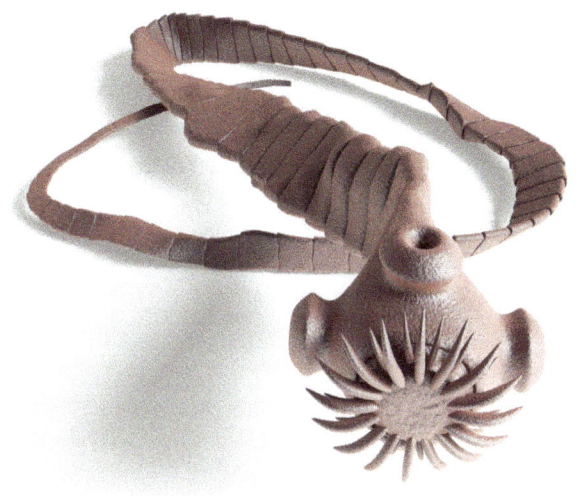

How long your cleanse and detox regimen lasts is totally up to you. Your parasite cleanse and detox could last from a week to a month or you may just want to make a lifestyle change altogether. You may just want to cleanse on the weekends it is totally up to you.

Detox Recipes

Have you have decided to eat a better and healthier diet this year? If yes, then you have come to the right place. Below you'll find recipes of 10 meals that can be prepared easily using whole, natural ingredients to detoxify your body. Let's try to stay away from processed foods for as long as we can, and opt for a nutrient-rich diet!

Avocado Egg Salad

Everyone will love this tasty avocado egg salad that uses egg yolks and lots of healthy fats from the avocado.

Ingredients:

Four chopped hard-boiled eggs.

Four chopped boiled egg whites.

One medium avocado. (Cut into half inch pieces)

Kosher salt-half teaspoon

Light mayonnaise – 1 tablespoon

Red wine vinegar- 2 tablespoons

Chopped chives- ½ tablespoon

Fat free plain yogurt- 1 tablespoon

A pinch of ground pepper

Directions:

Mix the avocado, egg yolks, yogurt, light mayo, vinegar, chives, salt and pepper in a bowl. Mash the mixture with a fork and then combine it with egg whites. Serve and enjoy!

Sweet Pea Juice

Sweet pea Juice is a deliciously refreshing juice which is loved by people of all ages! Serve it with lunch.

Ingredients:

A quarter cup of fresh cilantro

Half teaspoon of stevia powder

One large, peeled and segmented, orange

One cup of peeled peas (sugar snap)

Two large, cored and diced, apples

Directions:

Put all the ingredients in a blender and blend until they are liquefied. Pour into a serving glass, and serve chilled.

GF Ginger Pasta Salad

Even pasta can be included into your detox diet plan, it's quick and easy to make. Not only that, it is also mouth-watering!

Ingredients:

One pound gluten-free pasta

A quarter cup of finely chopped parsleys

1 Tablespoon of toasted pine nuts

Half cup of almond milk

A quarter cup of dried cranberries

1 tablespoon fresh ginger

A quarter tablespoon of white pepper (freshly ground)

A quarter tablespoon of sea salt

1 tablespoon of ground cinnamon

1 tablespoon of orange zest

Direction:

Boil the pasta as per the instructions of the package. Remove the pasta from heat when it is boiled, and pour cold water on it in a colander then transfer it to a large bowl. Add the remaining ingredients to the bowl and mix gently. Serve warm!

CREAMY BEAN DIP

Creamy Bean Dip is a great appetizer that can be prepared in just 15 minutes!

Ingredients:

A quarter teaspoon of sea salt

One tablespoon of fresh lemon juice

One clove of peeled and minced garlic

Two cans of drained and rinsed white beans

Quarter teaspoon of black pepper

Five tablespoons of extra virgin olive oil

2 tea spoons of balsamic vinegar

1 table spoon of fine chopped fresh basil

Directions:

Put all the ingredients in a food processor and pulse it until you get a smooth dip. Serve it fresh as an appetizer with your lunch!

TOMATOES WITH FRIED EGGS ON GARLIC TOAST

Tomatoes have numerous health benefits, and when they are cooked in olive oil they lower the risk of heart diseases. You can include tomatoes in your detox diet with this delicious lunch recipe!

Ingredients:

One clove of peeled garlic

2 tablespoons of Extra-virgin olive oil

Four large eggs

Freshly ground pepper

Coarse salt

Four small potatoes sliced in half

Toasted bread

Directions:

Heat oil in a frying pan on medium heat, crack eggs into it and let them cook undisturbed for two to three minutes until the whites are stable and set. Season the egg with spices and transfer into a plate.

Brush the cut sides of tomatoes with olive oil, and fry them in a frying pan on medium heat until they are charred. Transfer the two tomato halves to each toast and mash lightly with a spatula. Sprinkle spices on top, and place the fried eggs on top.

Serve hot with the peas juice mentioned above!

STEAMED BASS WITH FENNEL, PARSLEY, AND CAPERS

If you're feeling like having something exquisite then you'll really love this delicious fish recipe. If is both healthy and yummy.

Ingredients:

One tablespoon of rinsed capers

Half lemon juiced

Quarter medium white onion that has been sliced,

Half tablespoon sea salt

1 thinly sliced fennel bulb

A quarter cup of Italian parsley, chopped

Three tablespoons of extra virgin olive oil

Three to six ounces of striped bass portions

Chopped fresh parsley and additional olive oil for garnishing

Directions:

Pour water in a medium sauce pan up to one inch and add fennel, onion and lemon juice into it. Bring it to boil and then simmer for five minutes. Then remove the pan from heat, and add the bass portions seasoned with sea salt.

Sprinkle the pan with parsley and capers, and cover the pan. Simmer the pan until the fish becomes almost flaky. Finally, take a shallow bowl and place vegetables into the bottom and the bass on top of it. Sprinkle olive oil and parsley. Enjoy!

Detox Salad

Don't be fooled by the name, it's not as boring as it sounds. This colorful salad is wholesome, and delicious. You'll be craving for more after you finish your first bowl.

Ingredients:

Half cup raisins

One bunch Broccoli (stems removed)

Three cups of shredded carrots

One head cauliflower, (stems removed)

Pure maple syrup

Half cup sunflower seeds

Kelp (optional)

One cup currants

Half cup finely chopped parsley

Four to six tablespoons of fresh lemon juice to taste

Kosher salt, to taste

Pepper, to taste

Directions:

Finely chop broccoli, carrots and cauliflower and put in a large bowl. Put in sunflower seeds, raisins, currants, and parsley. Season the salad according to your taste and drizzle with maple syrup.

RAINBOW SALAD

Rainbow salad is a nutritious powerhouse. It is packed with health, I recommend eating it at least once a week. It's very easy to make.

Ingredients:

Two cups of dry rainbow Slaw

A small diced red bell pepper

Two cups chopped romaine

One Avocado

Salt and pepper to taste

Two table spoons of sesame seeds.

Directions:

Add romain, red pepper, and slaw in a large bowl and mix it together. Take out the salad in a plate and slice the avocado and put in the dishes. Sprinkle with spices and sesame oil. Enjoy!

BAKED SWEET POTATO WITH GREENS

If you're looking for a happy, hearty lunch then look no further! Simply bake your potatoes, and throw in a few spices and vegetables to get a delicious meal. If you are in a hurry, you can back your potatoes by microwaving them for about 6-8 minutes

Ingredients:

One tablespoon extra-virgin olive oil

One small onion sliced thinly

Two pricked sweet potatoes

One chopped and stemmed Swiss chard

Coarse salt

Lemon

One sliced avocado that has been divided

Cayenne

Directions:

Preheat the oven to 400 degrees and bake sweet potatoes until tender. It should take around 50 minutes. Heat oil in a large frying pan on medium heat and then add onions. Let them cook until they are tender and then add chard. Keep stirring until it becomes green and wilted. Season it with salt.

Serve by splitting potatoes and topping each piece with the greens and the half slides of avocado. Season them with salt, lemon, and cayenne. Enjoy.

Honey Greek Yogurt

Honey Greek Yogurt is delicious and healthy! It is also ready in a jiffy; you can serve it in lunch along with your main course.

Ingredients:

Two cups of Greek plain yogurt

A quarter tea spoon of vanilla extract

One teaspoon of ground cinnamon

Two tablespoons of silvered almonds

2 tablespoons of ground flax seeds

Directions:

Combine yogurt and vanilla extract in a bowl and mix them will. Add cinnamon, almond and flax seeds to the mixture. Serve chilled!

Have fun cooking!

Dinner on the Detox Diet doesn't have to be bland! Here are ten tasty recipes to help you eat smart and enjoy some delicious slimming dishes.

Carrot Bisque Deluxe. This delicately flavored soup makes a perfect light dinner for family. It serves four.

Ingredients

1½ lbs. carrots

1 large onion

1 clove garlic

¼ cup olive oil

½ tsp ginger

3 tsp curry powder

6 cups vegetable stock

Chopped parsley and chives to taste

½ cup fat-free sour cream

Directions

Peel and dice the carrots, onions, and garlic. Sauté in the hot olive oil until transparent. Add garlic, curry, ginger, and stock. Cover the pan and simmer until carrots are tender, about 25 minutes.

Uncover the pan and allow it to cool, then puree the soup in the blender. Adjust the seasoning with salt and pepper. Return to the pan and reheat. Serve with dollops of sour cream topped with chopped parsley and chives.

Ginger stir-fry. Make sure that your veggies are super-fresh when you prepare this delicious dish.

Ingredients

10 oz. rice noodles

2 tbsp. olive oil

Sweet pepper, any color

Fresh ginger (aim for a piece about ¾ in long

1 large or 3 small carrots

10 asparagus tips

4 oz. sugar snap peas

½ cup hoisin sauce

2 heads Bak Choi

7 scallions

Directions

Cut the pepper into thin strips. Peel, slice, and dice the ginger root. Cut the bak choi into 3-inch pieces. Slice the scallions. Prepare rice noodles according to package directions.

In hot oil, stir-fry the prepared vegetables for about 2 minutes. Add the hoisin sauce and ¼ cup water, and continue to stir-fry for about 5 minutes. Now drain the noodles, arrange them on a platter, and top with the vegetables. If you like, season with soy sauce.

Chicken and tomato dinner salad. This dish is quick to fix, especially if you have some leftover broccoli. Serves 4.

Ingredients

For the dressing:

2 tbsp. olive oil

1 clove garlic, chopped

1 tsp dried tarragon

For the chicken:

BONELESS CHICKEN BREASTS

1 tbsp. olive oil

1 cup cherry tomatoes

1 cup salad greens, torn into bite-size pieces

3 tbsp. sliced fresh scallions

1 oz. pine nuts

1 cup broccoli spears, cooked

Directions

Mix the dressing ingredients and set aside. Cut the chicken breasts into strips and fry the chicken in the oil until cooked through, about 10 minutes. Add the broccoli and tomatoes and stir for about one minute. Turn off the heat under the pan and pour in the salad dressing. Arrange salad greens in dish and top with the chicken and broccoli. Garnish with pine nuts.

Prawns Marsala. Lovely seafood in a rich sauce: what's not to love? This dish will serve 2 diners.

Ingredients

5 oz. tiger prawns, cooked and with shells and tails removed

1 ½ cup vegetable stock

1 tbsp. cornstarch

½ tsp salt

3 tbsp. olive oil

1 cup sliced mushrooms

1 clove garlic, chopped

½ cup Marsala wine

Directions

Mix the cornstarch with a bit of the stock. Bring the stock to a boil, add the cornstarch and salt, and let it thicken. Set aside. Sauté the mushrooms and garlic in the oil until light brown. Pour in the wine, add the thickened stock, and then the prawns.

Quick baked potato with tuna. For four servings bake four medium russet potatoes. Drain a can of solid white tuna, toss with 1 cup of diced basil-and-garlic tomatoes and 3 chopped scallions. Split the potatoes, top with the tuna mixture, heat under broiler until slightly browned.

CLAM ZITI WITH BROCCOLI. Serves four.

Ingredients

2 – 6 oz. cans chopped or minced clams

Salt, pepper, and parsley to taste

Lemon wedges

3 tbsp. olive oil

12 oz. ziti

3 cups chopped broccoli, cooked

1 large onion, chopped

8 oz. sliced mushrooms.

Directions

Heat the oil and sauté the onion and mushrooms until mushrooms are lightly brown and onions are translucent. Add undrained clams and broccoli. Turn heat to low. Meanwhile, cook pasta until al dente, and then drain. Toss the ziti with the clam sauce, season to taste with salt and pepper, and serve with chopped parsley and lemon wedges.

Taco Salad. Fill a salad bowl with chopped red-leaf lettuce, romaine, and a bit of cilantro. Add slices of tomato and avocado. Chop ½ cup of walnuts very fine, toss with cumin, coriander, chili powder to taste, and toss with the salad greens. Garnish with salsa.

Baked sweet potato. Bake four sweet potatoes in a 375 degree oven until tender, about 1 hour. Chop a whole tomato and a medium onion, and sauté in one tbsp. olive oil. Dress the potatoes with the tomato/onion mix, and top with avocado slices. Serves four.

Grilled chicken with veggies. You can enjoy this dish while eating al fresco. Arrange cubes of chicken breast, zucchini rounds, cherry tomatoes, and red pepper strips on skewers. Cook over the grill, basting with olive oil. Remove from skewers and garnish with sliced avocado and chopped parsley

WATER DETOX MADE EASY

Natural detoxification of your body has become increasingly popular.

With health and diet markets cornered with countless supplements, shakes, pills, and products, some of the most basic methods of keeping your body healthy and clean are forgotten in the mix.

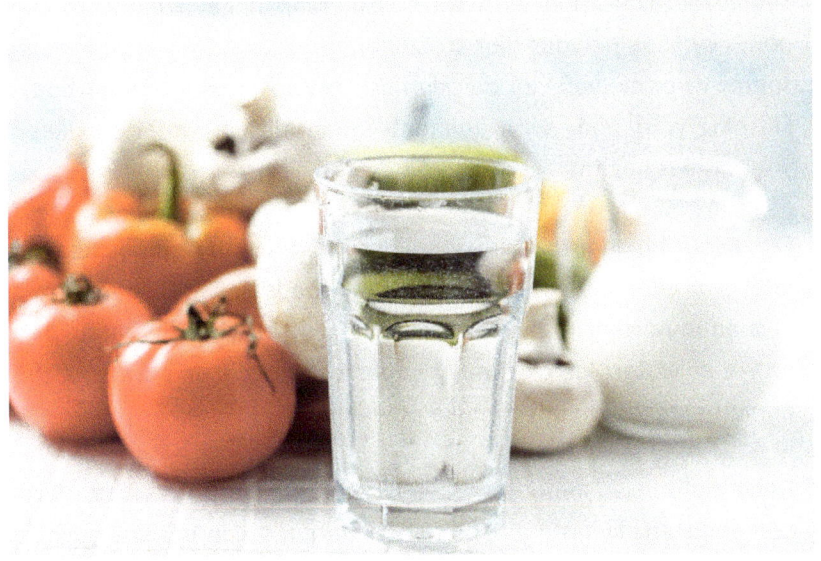

For centuries, it has been tried and tested, and each time the simplest foundation of life which is water, is recognized as the most important aspect to a healthy life. Without water after only a few short days, your body will begin to dehydrate and perish. Adequate hydration is imperative to staying healthy, vibrant, and energetic.

But even the most basic and fundamental element of water can give you the best and most absolute results when it comes to cleansing and detoxifying your body. It is recommended that the average human consume eight glasses of water at least eight ounces per day.

This recommendation is hardly and rarely met. As you allow your body to dehydrate, toxicity levels also build. This obviously harms the body as it saps your energy and causes general lethargy. If you do not eat healthily, such as too many fatty foods and carbohydrates, you will tend to build up more toxicity within your body.

Simple detoxification with water can reap huge benefits to the body. By keeping your diet strictly adhered to water as your main source of drink, you can quickly flush any toxins out of your body. Flushing your body with adequate quantities of water can keep your organs healthy.

From your bladder to your kidneys, good function requires healthy intake of adequate water and healthy foods as well. Your liver is also an important organ that relies heavily on your hydration and intake of water. It's extremely important to consume at least the minimum recommended intake of water.

Dehydration is sometimes unrecognizable until it's too late. Sometimes its symptoms don't show until it's also too late such as when you may get heatstroke. Being out in the heat for too extended a period of time without adequate water will lead definitively to dehydration and possibly heatstroke. These dangerous conditions can compromise the systems organs entirely. If left untreated, it can surely lead to major problems possibly even death.

Detoxifying with water is a very effective and inexpensive way to rehydrate, energize, and recharge your body. Flushing out toxins and substances that have accumulated by detoxification with water can increase your quality of life drastically.

Adding a citrus fruit such as a lemon to your water can also help with your diet by increasing the body's ability to cut fat. The benefits of water are endless.

By staying adequately hydrated and drinking plenty of water, you will retain and possibly your body's energy and health. The added benefit is the removal of those toxins that build up after we eat unhealthily and perhaps fail to exercise enough.

Detoxifying with water for certain specific substances, such as alcohol, can also speed up the process of purging the alcohol from your system and rendering you a quicker, smoother recovery.

Detoxifying your body with water is as simple as drinking adequate amounts throughout your daily regimen. The better hydrated you stay the healthier your body is on the inside. What that will do for you is reflect on the outside as well. Your skin, energy level, and vibrancy can be restored by simply detoxifying your body with water.

There are many ways you can introduce water detoxification into your life. None of them require any specific recipe or ingredient which may be the beauty behind the simplicity of water detoxification. It's as simple as drinking enough water throughout the day, everyday.

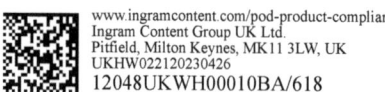